Alkaline Diet Guide

Lose Weight Quickly, Achieve Optimal Health, and Feel Energized with the Alkaline Diet and Alkaline Recipes

Emma Rose

Table of Contents

Introduction

I want to thank you and congratulate you for purchasing the book, "**Alkaline Diet Guide**: *Lose Weight Quickly, Achieve Optimal Health and Feel Energized with the Alkaline Diet and Alkaline Recipes*".

This book contains proven steps and strategies on how you can achieve a more efficient weight loss and at the same time, boost both your energy and health by simply changing the kind of food that you eat. Going Alkaline isn't a new method but for many, the process is still an uncharted road. Let this book be your guide.

Here you'll be provide with an easy to follow process. From start to finish, you'll find all that you need in order to get started as well as enough knowledge to take you to the next phase of the diet itself-- living a healthy, alkaline rich life.

Thanks again for purchasing this book, I hope you enjoy it! Please take some time to stop by and LIKE our Facebook page:

https://www.facebook.com/joypublishing

With gratitude,

Emma Rose

Chapter 1: What Is The Alkaline Diet?

In its basic sense, the alkaline diet (also known under other names such as the acid ash diet, alkaline ash diet and alkaline acid diet) is the belief that certain foods have a significant effect on both the pH and acidity of our body fluids such as blood or urine. With that in mind, it is said that by tweaking these, we can also make use of these food products to help treat certain diseases as well as prevent them. But that's not all-- it has also been said that keeping in line with this diet can also help you lose excess weight.

It's the kind of pitch that anyone would love-- and this is a fact further proven by the Hollywood celebrities who have tried the diet itself. Just take Victoria Beckham for example. But they aren't the only ones who can back up the diet's effectiveness when it comes to weight loss. It all goes back, way back to the time of our hunter-gatherer ancestor's diets.

This is what the Alkaline Diet is based upon, after all. That modern man's everyday diet has basically ruined our metabolic systems (along with other environmental factors), causing it to slow down and become inefficient when it comes to burning up fat from the food we eat. To help you understand that better, here's a quick summary of facts:

1. This "caveman" diet was based on animal foods and minimally (almost none at all) processed plants. However, as time progressed and agriculture became a main source of livelihood for man, the standard Western diet went through an immense change.

2. Grains aren't a typical part of our diet and our bodies, according to the Alkaline Guide, isn't meant to digest these. The same applies to milk, cheese and other

derivative products for these were only introduced after the man has learned to domesticate livestock.

3. Sugar and salt consumption rose towards the beginning of the Industrial revolution and in some way, our body never really got used to having too much of it-- way beyond what we can normally get from fruits and other plant food.

4. The diet we all have now is highly acidic and this causes numerous health problems, unsurprisingly. This is what the alkaline diet wishes to change, and basically wants to bring us back to what was more natural for us to consume. Basically resetting our metabolisms-- and making us fat burning "machines" just like our ancestors.

Now, all of that might sound a little complicated but the further we go, the easier it will be to understand. Let's start with acidic food and how it affects our bodies.

Almost all of the food products that we consume, once we have digested and metabolized it, would release either an alkaline base or an acid base into our blood. Grains, meat, shellfish, milk, poultry, cheese and salt all produce acid hence unbalancing the proper pH of our blood (which is slightly alkaline). This kind of diet, if continued and not counteracted by alkaline foods, can cause some serious side effects. Symptoms of a highly acidic diet include:

1. A lack of energy and a sensation of heaviness in your limbs. This can also include a loss of your psychic drive as well as physical tone. You might also feel depressed or an inability to cope.

2. You are more susceptible to different illnesses and infections.

3. You frequently feel cold and your body temperature has significantly lowered. You might also get frequent headaches or dizzy spells.

4. You have dry skin which also tends to experience irritations in areas where you sweat a lot. This is because your sweat has become highly acidic as well and if you have sensitive skin, you might feel slight burning sensations on it.

5. You might also experience stomach pains due to excess gastric acid or acid regurgitation. Ulcers and gastritis are also common symptoms associated with a highly acidic diet.

By switching up the food you regularly eat into something more alkaline, you would be able to avoid all of that and bring back the proper pH balance of your blood. Not to mention the fact that you'll also be helping your metabolism return to normal-- making it more efficient when it comes to burning up fat and using it for energy. That alone would hasten the process of weight loss for you.

Chapter 2: Benefits of the Alkaline Diet

Reading the previous chapter might have provided you with an insight as to how the diet works and what it is based upon. However, it does not provide you with any clue as to how it can benefit you-- other than the fact that it would help you lose weight and make your body more efficient when it comes to using the nutrients we get from the food we eat. In this chapter, we'll talk about the benefits and how that affects your overall health.

1. *Improved Energy Levels* – When it comes to your overall level of energy, one of the most important factors would be proper cell function. Basically, if your cells are not healthy then they won't be very effective when it comes to holding as well as transferring oxygen throughout your body. What this results to is fatigue and an absolute lack of energy.

Another factor would be body's pH level. It can significantly affect the cell's ability to provide ATP or adenosine triphosphate, this is also very important to the energy our body is capable of producing. The process of "making" it happens within a cell's mitochondria but if your pH level becomes too acidic, this is hindered. So if you've noticed a recent drop in your energy or if you've been feeling lethargic lately, you might want to look into the diet you've been indulging in. Chances are, the foods you consumed are highly acidic and are messing with the proper pH of your body.

2. *Improved Immune Function* – When your cells are healthy, they are more capable of absorbing the nutrients that your body requires. They are also more efficient when it comes to getting rid of waste products. However, should they be weakened, these functions are compromised as well. As a direct result of this, your

immune function is also threatened and you become more susceptible to different infections and different illnesses. This is among the many ill effects that a highly acidic diet can bring about. Cell damage is just the first of many in the process. So keep your cells healthy by making sure you eat the right stuff.

3. *Slower Aging* – As we have learned, subjecting your cells to highly acidic environment constantly will cause their efficiency to decrease a lot. This also results in its inability to quickly repair itself which leads to premature aging. This happens when the cells don't get enough oxygen and are rendered unable to rid themselves of damaging toxins. An alkaline diet certainly helps in this situation and would help you maintain healthy cells and a youthful appearance as well. Remember that healing your skin doesn't always start from the inside. Sometimes you have to look at the food you eat and make changes to ensure healthy skin.

4. *Reduced Pain and Inflammation* – Magnesium is one of the most important minerals that the body utilizes when it comes to controlling high levels of acid. So if you keep on eating a highly acidic diet, your body would then need to use more magnesium in order to neutralize it. Because of this, it can get depleted thus resulting to tissue and joint pain. Eating alkaline rich foods would help restore the lost magnesium and you'll be able to avoid all of the above without trouble.

5. *Weight Loss* – In changing the food that we eat, we are also able to reset our metabolisms and make it more efficient when it comes to burning food for fuel. The alkaline diet calls for more greens instead of animal protein and that small change alone can help significantly. Remember that our metabolism has a much harder time with animal protein and in time, it actually slows it down. You can fix and clean that up by switching to lighter but no less healthy food products.

The same kind our ancestors would have eaten but in proper balance this time. It's all about maintaining that and making sure that your body is still getting all of the nutrients that it needs to function better.

6. *Healthier Teeth and Gums* – You may not think much about this but a highly acidic diet can certainly affect the health of your gums and teeth. This is because bacteria grows at a much faster rate if your mouth is acidic and that could cause innumerable problems-- starting with bad breath to some serious gum disease. Of course, it also puts you at risk of experiencing tooth decay. An alkaline diet balances even the acids in your mouth so you can avoid experiencing all of that. Many people have noted a significant improvement in their oral health after switching to the diet program.

7. *Neutralizes Acid Imbalance* – An acid imbalance in the body can lead to numerous issues and as such, it should be treated immediately. Just think about the pain that ulcer or hyperacidity can cause. It can be paralyzing in some cases and might even require you to undergo surgeries just so the damage it has caused can be fixed. If you've ever experienced acid reflux then you also know how sick that feels and how much it burns the throat which can also lead to tissue damage as well. Needless to say, this isn't something that you can simply ignore. The best treatment for it isn't medication or surgery-- you don't even need to reach that stage if you simply make dietary and lifestyle changes.

8. *Lowers Risk Factors for Certain Diseases* – It has been said that eating a well-balanced alkaline diet can also help in lowering your risk for developing health problems such as colon cancer and type 2 diabetes. While studies are still being done on it, it's safe to say that the idea isn't too farfetched considering the fact that you'll be switching to healthier foods during the diet and would also need to drop certain bad habits

9

such as smoking if you're to really continue living an alkaline life.

9. *Improve your Heart's Overall Health* – Again, studies are still being done on this but many have said that it did help them improve their cardiovascular health. This is mainly attributed to the fact that the program highly encourages people to eat a well-balanced diet comprised of both greens and meat. It isn't about restricting yourself but instead, it guides you towards finding a plan that works for your needs and that of your health. Cutting back on red meat is one of its core ideas and that alone already helps in preventing certain heart-related issues brought on by high cholesterol.

10. *Detoxification* – Let's talk free radicals and how these things can really take your body for a loop. They are everywhere. In the food that we eat and in our environment so they're not very easy to avoid. Instead, we have to build up a strong defense against them and regularly detoxify our bodies so that they get flushed out long before they have any chance of ruining our cells. However, not a lot of people really pay attention to this and unless they feel something weird happening to their bodies, would still continue on with their bad diet and everyday habits.

If you want to live a longer, healthier life then detoxification is one of the key things you'll need. Eating an alkaline rich diet is one of the biggest steps you can take because it promotes detoxifying food products as part of the meal plans. Couple that with a regular exercise routine and you'll be able to clean up your body in no time. You'll feel its effects almost instantaneously too. More energy, refreshed, brighter skin and eyes, a better ability to concentrate-- those are just a few of the benefits it can provide you with.

Chapter 3: Alkaline Food List

The thing about acidic and alkaline foods is that you can't tell which is which at first glance. Some foods might appear or taste like they could be acidic but are actually alkaline, such is the case of citrus fruits. It is the way our body reacts to a particular food product that ultimately determines whether it's acidic or alkaline.

Now, nearly all vegetable, fruits, nuts, seeds and herbs have alkalizing effects on our bodies though the degrees at which they do tend to vary. Just take tea for example, almost all varieties save for black tea are all alkaline. Rule of thumb is that foods that are not processed and remain closest to their natural state tend to be more alkaline than most. This means that any kind of *processed food such as grains, dairy and fast food tend to be acidic.*

Note that pesticides are actually known to be acid-forming so chose organic when it comes to your fruits and vegetables. Then you have your legumes and beans-- a vegetarian's main source of protein-- which are also acidic. With that said, however, don't eliminate acidic foods from your diet completely. Just make sure that you balance everything well. 60-80% alkaline to 20-40% acidic foods should be just right.

To give you something a bit more specific, here's a quick rundown of the most commonly eaten alkaline foods.

Alkalizing Vegetables

- alfalfa, beet greens, broccoli, barley greens, cabbage, celery, carrot, chard greens, cucumber, dandelions, edible flowers, dulce, fermented veggies, eggplant, green beans, garlic, green peas, lettuce, kohlrabi, kale, mustard greens, mushrooms, parsnips, onions, peas, pumpkins, peppers, nightshade veggies, rutabaga, radishes, spirulina, sea veggies, sprouts, spinach, sweet potatoes, watercress, tomatoes, wild greens and wheat grass.

- dandelion root, daikon, maitake, kombu, reishi, nori, wakame, umeboshi and shitake.

- avocado, apricot, apple, berries, banana, sour cherries, cantaloupe, fresh coconut, currants, figs, dates, grape fruit, grapes, lime, lemon, honeydew melon, nectarine, muskmelons, orange, pineapple, pear, peach, raspberries, raisins, rhubarb, tomato, tangerine, strawberries, umeboshi plum, tropical fruits and watermelon.

- millet, chestnuts, almonds, fermented tofu, fermented tempeh, whey protein powder, stevia (sweetener).

Now, if you're a beginner and have been eating a highly addictive consumerist diet for most of your life then making the switch can be much harder than you think. The foremost reason for this is that your body would eventually crave its usual food and you might end up binge eating because of it too. In order to avoid all of that, pace yourself and start bit by bit. Here are some of the most alkaline forming foods that you can easily work into your everyday meals. Think of them as stepping stones as you slowly transition into a mostly alkaline diet.

1. *Root Vegetables* – Because of the healing nature of these foods, they are often used in traditional Chinese medicine to help with different illnesses. These are rich in vitamins and minerals, more than your average vegetable making it a great addition to any diet. So if you're looking to start simple, try root vegetables as

they can also be cooked in different ways. The best bit? They are quite filling so you'll feel satiated after.

2. *Cruciferous Vegetables* – These would include the veggies that many people love. Broccoli, cauliflower and cabbage are just prime examples of this variety. While they are already typically included in your daily diet, you can do more by utilizing them in different ways. As dips or as garnishes, the more you consume of these the better.

3. *Garlic* – When it comes to foods that promote overall health, garlic is among those at the top. It is alkaline-forming but also helps improve heart and immune health. It cleanses the liver and lowers blood pressure while fighting off disease. While it does have a strong smell, there are a number of ways to prepare it which should help with reducing it.

4. *Cayenne Peppers* – This contains enzymes that are actually essential when it comes to our endocrine function-- besides the fact that it is also one of the most alkalizing foods. Not only that, it comes with a rich supply of vitamin A and antibacterial properties which is great if you're looking to detoxify and get rid of free radical in your body.

5. *Lemons* – These are the most alkalizing foods available, and they are also natural disinfectants that are capable of healing wounds. It also energizes the liver and can provide immediate relief if you're experiencing hyperacidity. So a glass of freshly squeezed lemon before or after every meal is a great way of incorporating it into your daily diet. Eating the fruit itself is also great-- if you can stand how sour some of it can be.

Alright, so now that you've got some idea of which foods to pick and which ones you should eat less off, let's move to applying all of it to your daily diet.

Chapter 4: Alkaline Diet Recipes

Let's begin with something easy and quick to prepare. Using alkaline-forming ingredients, these should provide you with the energy you need for the day.

Spelt Porridge

Ingredients:

- 1 cup of filtered water
- 1/3 cup of flaked spelt
- Powdered stevia or agave for sweetening
- Cinnamon to taste
- 2-3 tablespoons of cranberries or cherries (dried)
- ¼ teaspoon of vanilla

Toppings: hemp nuts, raw nuts, blueberries, hazelnut and hemp milk.

Procedure:

1. Combine your first 6 ingredients and allow it to simmer for at least 3 to 4 minutes before transferring it to a shallow bowl.

2. Once done, sprinkle your toppings all over it.

3. Add your non-dairy milk (almond or hazelnut would work too).

4. Serve warm.

Power Smoothie

Ingredients:

- 1 ¼ of coconut water
- ½ cup of unsweetened almond milk
- A cup of frozen blueberries
- 2/3 cup of frozen raspberries
- 2 tablespoons of agave or stevia
- 1 avocado, sliced
- 3 tablespoons of fresh coconut meat
- ½ a teaspoon of super greens powder
- 4 tablespoons of raw hemp nuts
- 2 tablespoons of omega 3 oil

Procedure:

1. Combine all of your ingredients in a blender.

2. Mince your raspberries and add some more coconut water if you think the consistency needs it.

3. Blend well until it becomes thick and creamy.

4. Yields 4 cups.

Spelt and Vanilla Vegan Pancakes

Ingredients:

- 1 cup of light spelt flour
- 1/8 teaspoon of fine Himalayan salt
- 2 tablespoon of aluminum free baking powder
- 1 cup of almond milk
- 1 tablespoon of maple syrup or stevia
- 1 ½ teaspoon of alcohol free vanilla
- 2 tablespoons of cold pressed sunflower oil
- Coconut oil for greasing

Procedure:

1. Measure all of your dry ingredients in one bowl and the wet ones into a separate one.

2. Give each a stir before combining. Make sure it's mixed well and evenly.

3. Set this aside for at least 5 minutes and allow it to rise.

4. While waiting, prepare your open pan and brush on ¼ teaspoon of coconut oil on it, keeping the heat low.

5. Spoon your batter into this, forming 3 small pancakes. Cook for 3 minutes or until each side become golden.

Hot Chocolate with Coconut Milk

Ingredients:

- ½ cups of unsweetened almond milk
- 10 tablespoons of coconut milk powder
- 1 ½ cup of filtered water
- 6 drops of stevia
- 5 tablespoon of raw cacao powder
- cinnamon
- marshmallows
- 1 ½ tablespoon of agave

Procedure:

1. Using a medium sized sauce pan, mix all of your ingredients together.

2. Make sure you keep the heat on low and whisk until you remove all the lumps.

3. Adjust the sweetness if preferred and serve it topped with marshmallows.

Spring Pea and Edamame Bread Spread

Ingredients:

- 1 ½ cup of fresh peas
- 1 ½ cup of edamame beans
- ½ teaspoon of salt
- 1/3 cup of extra virgin olive oil + some extra
- 3 stems of fresh mint
- Juice from one lime
- Lime Zest

Procedure:

1. Place your edamame beans in boiling water for about 4 minutes until it becomes bright green.

2. Removes them and run the beans under cold water.

3. Repeat the same for your peas except only leave them in for a minute.

4. Once done, place both in a food processor and combine until it gets evenly mixed. Don't puree completely.

5. Add some seasoning and serve in a bowl. A drizzle of olive oil and mint leaf garnish should top it off nicely.

6. Now that you've got easy to prepare recipes for your everyday breakfast, let's talk lunch. Fast foods are definitely part of your options so, what to do? Prepare it beforehand and take it with you!

Raw Zucchini Noodles with Pesto

Ingredients:

- 6 pieces of 8 inch zucchinis, peeled
- 1 cup of basil leaves
- Celtic sea salt
- 3 tablespoons of raw hemp hearts
- ¼ cup of pine nuts or raw cashews
- 1 clove of garlic, crushed
- ¼ cup of olive oil

Procedure:

1. Using your spiral slicer, trim the ends of your zucchini in order to make it line up evenly. Slowly wind it and carefully collect the spaghetti like noodles that would be pushing through the openings on the blade.

2. For fettuccine like noodles, (and if you have no spiral slicer) you can use a simple peeler. Just be careful and mind the thickness.

Pesto Sauce:
1. Combine your olive oil, basil, garlic, nuts and sea salt in a blender. Combine this until you achieve the right consistency. Add more oil if needed.

2. Toss this with your noodles and serve as is to keep noodles nice and crunchy.

Mini Roasted Veggie Skewers with Garlic Basil Dip

Ingredients:

- 1 sweet white onion
- 2 red peppers
- 3 zucchinis
- 3 cloves of crushed garlic
- 12 cherry tomatoes
- ¼ cup of olive oil
- Sea salt
- 12 pieces of skewers

For the dip:
- 2 cloves of garlic
- 1 cup of zucchini
- ½ a cup of extra virgin olive oil
- ½ cup of raw pistachio nuts
- 16 basil leaves
- ½ teaspoon of sea salt

Procedure:

1. Preheat your oven to 400F.

2. Combine our oil and garlic, set this aside.

3. Skewer your veggies, make sure there's a uniform pattern. Set aside.

4. Baste this well with the garlic oil, spreading the garlic bits onto your vegetable pieces.

5. Sprinkle some sea salt over it.

6. Roast for about 15 minutes.

7. For your dip, simply mix all of your dip ingredients in a blender/food processor until it becomes creamy. Add more olive oil if needed.

Sprouted Grain Wrap with Chipotle Dip

Ingredients:

- 1 peeled parsnip
- 2 medium sized beets
- 1 yellow beet
- 1 large sweet potato
- 4 tablespoons of olive oil
- 1 teaspoon salt
- Mixed greens
- 6 sprouted grain tortilla wraps
- Fresh pea shoots
- Chipotle Dip

Procedure:

1. Toss all of your veggies with oil and salt but keep your red beets separate.

2. Once done, spoon these into your baking sheet, sprinkling the red beets on top. Make sure it's parchment lined.

3. Roast this in a preheated oven (350 degrees) for about 25 minutes until it becomes slightly tender. Remove and allow to cool.

4. Over your wrap pile your greens and spoon some of the roasted roots down its center. Add some of your chipotle dip on top before sprinkling some of the pea shoots.

5. Serve with extra dip and some avocado.

Rainbow Salad with Avocado and Meyer Lemon Dressing

Ingredients:

- Baby spinach and arugula greens
- 1 yellow beet
- 2 carrots
- 6 slices of yellow pepper
- ¼ red onion
- Pea shots
- Micro greens or sprouts
- 1 avocado
- Chopped pistachios

Dressing:
- 1 avocado
- 2 lemons
- 1 ½ teaspoon of red onion
- 6 fresh dill
- 6 basil leaves
- 1/8 teaspoon of sea salt
- 1/3 cup cold pressed extra virgin olive oil
- 3 drops of stevia

Procedure:

1. Prepare your serving bowls.

2. In each of them place a generous amount of your arugula.

3. Top this with beets and surround that with other veggies. Make sure that everything is layered properly.

4. Add your micro greens, pea shoots and top this with your pistachios.

5. For the dressing, simply process all of the ingredients in a blender. Make sure it reaches a creamy consistency before pouring it in a separate container.

Raw Cranberry Pie to Go

Ingredients:

- 1 organic pear
- 2 cups of raw organic cranberries
- ¼ wedge of orange (keep the skin)
- Juice from half an orange
- ½ cup of raw almonds
- 6 dates
- ½ cup of raw pecans
- ¼ teaspoon of cinnamon
- 1/8 teaspoon allspice
- 1/8 teaspoon ground cloves
- 2 tablespoon of maple syrup
- ½ a teaspoon of vanilla
- 1 cup of untoasted buckwheat

Procedure:

For the base:
1. Soak your buckwheat using filtered water for half an hour. Rinse and drain properly.

2. Combine this with ¼ teaspoon of cinnamon and the orange juice. Add your maple syrup and half a teaspoon of vanilla. Set this aside.

For the filling:
1. Using your food processor, mix your cranberries, your orange, dates, a teaspoon of cinnamon, cloves, all spice and half and teaspoon of vanilla.

2. Make sure this is blended well then set aside.

For the pie topping:

1. Place 2 dates, pecans, almonds and ¼ teaspoon of cinnamon in a food processor.

2. Blend until it becomes crumbly.

3. Now fill your jar layer by layer. Buckwheat bottom, then 2 scoops of the cranberry mixture and topped with the nut crumbles.

4. Top this with some fresh cranberry and seal the lid.

Dairy Free Cherry, Avocado and Coconut Ice Cream

Ingredients:

- 2 cups of cherries + 6 more, finely chopped
- ½ of a large avocado
- 1 400ml organic full fat coconut milk
- 1/3 cup of cashews
- 10 soft dried dates
- Juice of half a lemon
- 2/3 cup of filtered water
- 1/3 cup of cashews, soaked and drained
- 2 tablespoon agave syrup
- 2 tablespoon beet juice (for color)
- Finely chopped dark chocolate

Procedure:

1. Using a high speed blender, combine 2 cups of cherries, avocado, coconut milk, water, cashews, dates and lemon juice.

2. Blend this until it becomes creamy. Taste it for sweetness before adding your agave.

3. Stir your chocolate and chopped cherries into this mixture.

4. Transfer this to your ice cream maker and follow the instructions.

5. You can also choose to freeze this overnight.

6. Garnish with a few more chopped cherries before serving.

Aioli Fries

Ingredients:

- 1 Tablespoon of chili powder
- ½ Teaspoon of lemon juice
- 1 Tablespoon olive oil
- ½ Teaspoon sea salt
- 2 large sweet potatoes, sliced into fries

Aioli

- 1 avocado, scooped out
- 1 ½ Tablespoons parsley
- ¼ Tablespoon lemon juice
- ¼ Garlic clove
- 4 Teaspoons cumin
- Pinch sea salt & pepper
- ½ Tablespoons of olive oil

Procedure:

1. Begin by chopping your sweet potato into long strips in a cube shape, approximately 1cm. Try to make the ends even as if they are too thin they are more prone to burning.

2. Take your olive oil, chili powder, lemon juice and salt to liberally sprinkle over the top of your potatoes. Toss the potatoes to make sure they are coated all over.

3. Line your baking tray with baking paper and place your potatoes on the tray. Make sure the potatoes are evenly spaced as they will crisp better if they are not in contact with their neighbors.

4. Bake for 15 minutes at around 200 degrees before turning the potatoes and returning them to the oven for another 15 minutes.

5. While you're waiting for the potatoes to cook place the ingredients for your aioli into a mixer and blend until smooth. Sprinkle with paprika and season with pepper if you wish.

6. Take the potatoes out of the oven and let them stand for five minutes before serving.

Savory Bake

Ingredients:

- 2 Eggs, large
- 1 Cup egg whites
- ¼ Cup parmesan cheese
- ½ Cup cheddar cheese, shredded
- 1 Tablespoons onion (garlic) powder
- ¼ Teaspoon salt
- ¼ Teaspoon black pepper, ground
- ¼ Teaspoon cumin
- ½ Cup quinoa, cooked
- 1 Cup broccoli, coarsely chopped
- ¼ Cup parsley, chopped
- Cooking spray

Procedure:

1. Start by preheating your oven to around 350 and use your cooking spray to cover a non-stick muffin tin making sure you get both the sides and bottom.

2. Wisk up your eggs and egg whites. Add in the cheeses. Stir and add in the onion, salt, pepper and as much cumin as you feel you want according to the spiciness you prefer. About an eighth to a quarter of a tablespoonful should be more than enough.

3. Now add in your quinoa, parsley, spring onions, broccoli and mix.

4. Use your finished mixture to fill your muffin tin. You should aim to fill about three quarters of each muffin place.

You can crisp the tops by sprinkling some extra cheese on top if you desire.

5. Baking should take between 15-20 minutes and the muffins should be left to cool for around 10 mins. They are best served fresh out the oven

Green Power Shake

Ingredients:

- 1 Cucumber
- 2 Tomatoes
- 1 Avocado
- 1 Handful of kale
- ½ Lemon
- 1 Red pepper
- 1 Teaspoon vegetable stock
- 2 Heads of broccoli

Procedure:

1. Make sure to wash all the vegetable thoroughly and then chop up your tomatoes, pepper and avocado. Use about 75ml of warm water to dissolve your vegetable stock before placing your stock and avocado into a mixer.

2. Add the tomato, peppers and cucumbers next and blend into a liquid.

3. Add your broccoli, lemon and kale and blend until everything is mixed through before serving.

Chai Vanilla Porridge

Ingredients:

- 4 Cups of water
- ½ Teaspoon all spice
- 2 Teaspoons ground nutmeg
- 2 Cups of semi skimmed milk
- Rind of a lime
- 2 Vanilla bean pods
- 2 Cups of organic dry quinoa

Procedure:

1. Prepare your quinoa by measuring 1 cup and straining it using a fine mesh. Use cool water for up to 2 minutes and use your hand to help rinse through the quinoa by rubbing it and moving it around the strainer.

2. You should then add a splash of olive oil to a saucepan and bring to a medium heat before adding your quinoa. Let the water evaporate and watch the quinoa toast for nearly a minute.

3. Use 2 cups of water to stir the mixture and then bring it to the boil. Lower the heat to a minimum and cook for around quarter of an hour whilst covering the pan. Without removing the cover let it stand for five minutes.

4. Once your quinoa is cooked stir in your all spice, nutmeg and add milk with your vanilla pods. Warm through and you can also sprinkle some nuts of your choice across the top, we recommend ground almonds onto the top with your lime rind.

Mexican Gluten Free Wraps

Ingredients:

- 4 Gluten Free Tortilla Wraps (we recommend Udi's Gluten Free Tortillas)
- 1 Tin of kidney beans
- 2 Avocados
- 2 Pink Grapefruit
- A Sprinkling of walnuts
- 2 Tablespoons of hoisin sauce
- 4 Tomatoes
- 1 Red onion
- A few handfuls of watercress to garnish

Procedure:

1. First you'll want to create your tortilla bowls, set your oven to 180 and pop your tortillas over a medium sized bowl. Don't push them against the bowl to harshly, gently does it. Leave your tortillas for about 9 minutes until they've crisped up and retain the bowl shape. When they're ready, leave them to the side to cool.

2. In the meantime chop up your onions, tomatoes and add your beans. Add the hoisin sauce into the mix and toss. To make sure everything is nice and cool pop the mix into fridge while you move onto the next bit.

3. Peel and slice your avocado along with the grapefruit. Chop up your almonds as finely as you can.

4. Take the rest of your ingredients out of the fridge, mix it all together and pop it in your tortilla bowls. Garnish with watercress.

Butter Bean Sweet Potato Curry

Ingredients:

- 1 Tablespoon of vegetable oil
- ½ Small red onion
- ½ Clove garlic, chopped
- ½ Tablespoon chopped ginger
- 1 Tablespoon cumin
- 1 Tablespoon of garam masala
- 1 Cup chicken stock
- ½ Cup canned diced tomato
- 1 medium sweet potato, small dice
- Salt and freshly ground black pepper, to taste
- 2/3 Cup quinoa
- ½ Cup kidney beans
- Juice of 1/2 lime

Procedure:

1. It is best to add vegetable oil to a large saucepan over a medium heat, however if you're looking to cut down on the calories we would recommend the Fry-Light cooking spray. Take your ginger, garam masala, cumin and onions and throw them into the pan. It should take a little less than five minutes to cook, gently stirring it while it heats.

2. Turn up the heat a little and add the vegetable stock, tomatoes, kidney beans and sweet potatoes. Add a little salt and pepper for seasoning if desired.

3. Bring the pan to the boil before leaving the vegetables to simmer. Stir the mixture and add in the quinoa. Cover your saucepan and leave the mixture the simmer for 20 minutes.

4. Check the mixture to see if the potatoes have softened and cook for another five minutes or so if they haven't. Feel free to add any remaining stock if the heat has dried out the vegetables too much.

5. Stir in your spinach and then serve with a smattering a lime juice.

Stuffed Sweet Potatoes

Ingredients:

- 4 Medium sized sweet potatoes
- 4 Tablespoons almond butter
- 1 Clove garlic grated
- ½ Cup of water
- 1 Cup Broccoli florets
- 2 Red bell pepper cubed
- 2-3 Sprigs of Oregano, fresh
- ½ Teaspoon caraway seeds
- 2-3 Sprigs of Tarragon, fresh
- Pinch of salt
- Optional: ¼ to ½ Cup Feta Cheese

Procedure:

1. Pre-heat oven to 175°C 350°F.

2. Using just over half the almond butter cover your sweet potato and add a pinch of salt. Cook for approximately 45 minutes or until the potato turns soft.

3. Remove the potato from the oven and cut it open lengthways. Be careful not to rip the skin further as you open it and remove the insides. Put the flesh into a separate bowl.

4. Using a frying pan heat up the remaining almond butter along with the grated garlic and caraway seeds. Cook for a minute to a minute and a half. Now add half of the water and add your peppers, broccoli and parsley. Leave to cook for another 2 minutes.

5. Add a little water to your potatoes and your tarragon whilst using you salt to season.

6. Scoop your mixture back into the skins of your potatoes and garnish with herbs. If you're feeling super hungry feta cheese would make tasty addition to the top of the dish.

Almond Pancakes

Ingredients:

- 1 Cup Almond flour
- 2 Eggs
- 2 Tablespoon Olive Oil
- 1 Teaspoon Sea Salt
- 2 Cups Water
- 6 Tablespoons Olive Oil

Procedure:

1. Add all of your ingredients together in the mixer and leave them for 1-2 minutes until smooth. Alternatively mix your own way with flour, eggs and oil in a bowl. Add the salt before slowly adding the water. Mix until smooth for about 4 minutes.

2. Use cooking spray to cover your pan before gently pouring in the mixture. Make sure to flip both sides of the mixture when you feel the pan becoming hot.

Ginger Pumpkin Dessert

Ingredients:

- 2 Large egg yolks
- 0.1 lbs Caster sugar or granulated
- 1 Tablespoons dark rum
- ¼ Cup Orange juice
- 1 Tin solid-pack pumpkin puree (0.46 lbs)
- 1 Teaspoons pumpkin pie spice
- Pinch fine salt
- 1 Cup Double cream
- 0.06 lbs Chopped crystallized ginger

Procedure:

1. Fill a saucepan with water, around 2cm and use a medium heat to allow it to simmer

2. Place the sugar, orange juice, egg yolk and sugar into a mixing bowl. It is important that the bowl can withstand heat as you will need to place the bowl over the saucepan later. Now beat together the ingredients until the mixture starts to foam.

3. Once the mixture is nice and light you should settle the bowl over your saucepan. The bowl shouldn't touch the water. Whisk the mixture for another minute or two until the eggs are thick.

4. Take the bowl off the saucepan and beat in the pumpkin, spice and a smattering of salt. You should continue to mix in the ingredients until they have cooled. Once the mixture has cooled take about half of the ginger and stir it in to the mix.

5. Using a new bowl whip up the double cream until it starts to spike up. Fold the cream into your mixture.

6. Now divide the mixture evenly between four bowls. If you use deep wine glasses you can fill these instead for a nice touch. Use the rest of the ginger to sprinkle over the top of each bowl.

7. The mixture should be left to chill for at least two hours but we would recommend covering with Clingfilm and leaving the mixture overnight.

Poached Eggplant

Ingredients:

- 1 Eggplant, cut into quarters lengthways
- 2 Cups vegetable broth
- 2 Red chili, cut into quarters lengthways
- 2 Garlic cloves, smashed
- 4 Dates, roughly chopped
- 1 Inch Ginger, grated
- 1/2 Tablespoon sesame oil
- 1 Tablespoon sesame seeds, toasted
- 2 Spring onions, trim ends and slice
- 1/2 Lime, cut into wedges

Procedure:

1. Take your vegetable broth and pour into a pot large enough to mix the ingredients in. Add to the pot your chili, garlic and dates.

2. Bring your pot to the boil before adding your eggplant. After you've added the eggplant let the pot simmer on a low heat for about 20 minutes. Make sure to turn over your eggplant about half way through.

3. After 20 minutes remove the eggplant and set it to the one side.

4. Now reduce your broth after removing the lid. Do this until you can see the mixture thicken and then add ginger, cooking for a further minute.

5. After a minute take your broth and sieve it into a bowl. Take the remaining liquid and add your sesame oil.

6. To serve, take your sauce and pour it over your eggplant. Use your spring onions, lime and sesame seeds to garnish.

So there you have it, some easy to follow recipes that would surely infuse some alkaline into your daily diet. The best bit is that these recipes are actually heart friendly and won't add unwanted calories into your system. If you're trying to lose some weight, they're still perfectly fine to have. Just make note of ingredients that you might be allergic with and switch it to ones that you know are safe for you to eat.

We hope these recipes could serve as the basis for ones that you'll be creating for yourself!

Conclusion

Thank you again for purchasing *"**Alkaline Diet Guide***: Lose Weight Quickly, Achieve Optimal Health and Feel Energized with the Alkaline Diet and Alkaline Recipes"*!

I hope this book was able to help you to better understand how the Alkaline Diet works and how it can significantly benefit you when it comes to losing weight as well as staying healthy and energized.

The next step is to take what you have learned and put it into action. Try the diet and see how it improves your health; find out how it benefits you overall. Keep in mind that the only way you can truly test these things out is not by reading and judging it through that. Putting it to the test and experiencing it is the only way you'll know if it's the right one for you.

Remember, this isn't just a simple diet trend. *It's a lifestyle change for the better!*

In addition, please remember to check out our Facebook page in order to find other resources and upcoming promotions:

https://www.facebook.com/joypublishing

With sincere thanks,

Emma Rose

Preview Of "Paleo Desserts: Satisfy Your Sweet Tooth With Over 100 Quick and Easy Paleo Dessert Recipes and Paleo Baking Recipes"

Introduction

I want to thank you for purchasing the book, *"Paleo Desserts: Satisfy Your Sweet Tooth With Over 100 Quick and Easy Paleo Dessert Recipes and Paleo Baking Recipes"*.

This book contains 100 Paleo dessert and baking recipes on how to prepare delectable desserts without sacrificing your health.

All my life I've had a sweet tooth. I would even go as far as to say that I had a sugar addiction! Over the last few years my sugar addiction got worse: I had dessert multiple times a day and every day (I guess being a Foods teacher didn't help much). I would joke with people by telling them that I had my servings of vegetables for the day in chocolate...except, I still didn't have the vegetables. It got pretty bad. I knew I hated eating that much dessert but I couldn't stop. I would eat one FerrerroRocher and then go back for another. As I walked back to the treats, I would pass the mirror and think to myself, "I don't need to have this chocolate. But, ah, what the heck, I don't care." In the end, I'd have about 6 FerrerroRochers in addition to the other treats I had earlier that day.

Finally, I had to take the huge tray of FerrerroRochers to school to give to my students on Valentine's Day. There was no way I could eat the other 30 myself. Eating all this sugar caused a huge war within me. I knew that my extreme sugar eating was unhealthy for me but I didn't want to stop. I loved it too much. As a result, I wrestled between the ideal of where I wanted to be and the reality of where I was. I knew I had the discipline to say no to other things, so why couldn't I say no to chocolate?

I eventually came to the point where I was starting to get fed up with not feeling well. I had a lot of chronic pain in my neck and I was constantly tired. I knew that sugar was irritating the problem and causing inflammation in my body. At was starting to reach the breaking point. Ultimately, I chose to go off of sugar for at least three weeks to break the habit I had created for myself. It was seriously a miracle to stay consistent with my goal because I really didn't want to give up my favorite desserts.

Shortly after my decision to go off of sugar, I had a miscarriage. Experiencing the loss catapulted me into a massive journey to find health and proper nutrition. I did a live blood analysis with a naturopath to discover what was contributing to the terrible ways I was feeling. Seeing all the garbage I had in my blood forced me to go off of dairy, corn, oats, and wheat. I was left wondering, "What the heck am I going to eat? That stuff is in everything!"

Consequently, I stumbled upon the Paleo diet. It was the most relevant diet to what I was trying to accomplish. I was able to find things to eat for breakfast, lunch and dinner. But desserts were a whole other story. I felt like something was missing and I couldn't put my finger on it. The best I could come up with was apple slices dipped in almond butter: hardly satisfying. Paleo desserts ended up being the by-product of my search to find something, anything that I could enjoy.

I encourage you to make that switch to healthier and happier desserts with the hundred delicious and irresistible recipes presented in this book. You don't need to follow the same extremity that I did. But if you are taking the Paleo diet seriously, then you may find the same void of sweets in your life too. Cutting out all the processed foods and going back to the basics really does clear up the body and help it function better. I've seen the changes in my own life as hard as it's been to make those changes. You, too, can make the changes necessary and still have your sweets along the way!

Thank you again for purchasing this book. I hope you enjoy the recipes. Experiment with them and make substitutions to suit your needs.

Chapter 1

Brief History of Paleo Diet

The Sweet Effects

Why do you love sweet food? Why do you crave for more of that dessert so much? Your anatomy would tell you that sweet foods would cause the release of dopamine in the part of the brain that is associated with motivation and reward. Not only that, but studies show that sweets also produce an increased level of serotonin. Serotonin gives you that feeling of happiness and wellbeing. That's why it is better to give a box of chocolates when you want the person to be in a good mood.

Unfortunately, the quote you can't have your cake and eat it too applies here. The bad effects that sugar brings are common knowledge. The number one disease is diabetes. People are aware of diabetes and its complications. That is why even when you intensely crave for that delicious dessert, you try to control your urges and settle for nothing instead. Well, that is if your self-control is in good condition. More often than not, people would rather risk the medical condition and eat that sweet thing with all their heart.

I have had many slip ups in my own life. I went two months without chocolate...can you believe it? Then Easter came. I found that if I gave myself an inch, I would take a mile. Eating chocolate quickly got out of control. I rebelled because I was strict for so long. You may find yourself in the same situation and find it hard to balance the sugar cravings. Once the sugar cravings are there, your body craves more and then a vicious cycle begins.

Check out the rest of "Paleo Desserts: Satisfy Your Sweet Tooth With Over 100 Quick and Easy Paleo Dessert Recipes and Paleo Baking Recipes" on Amazon.

Or go to: http://amzn.to/1lZNcVI

Check Out My Other Books

Below you'll find some of my other books also available on Amazon and Kindle. Search for these titles on the Amazon website to find them.

Paleo Free Diet Guide for Beginners: Over 50 Paleo Free Recipes for Optimal Health & Fast Weight Loss

Paleo Desserts: Satisfy Your Sweet Tooth With Over 100 Quick & Easy Paleo Dessert Recipes & Paleo Baking Recipes

Raw Food Diet Guide: Lose Weight Quickly, Achieve Optimal Health & Feel Energized with the Raw Food Diet & Raw Food Recipes

Clean Eating Guide: Lose Weight Quickly, Achieve Optimal Health & Feel Energized with Clean Eating For Busy Families & Clean Eating Recipes

Alkaline Diet Guide: Lose Weight Quickly, Achieve Optimal Health & Feel Energized with the Alkaline Diet & Alkaline Recipes

Coconut Flour Recipes for Optimal Health & Quick Weight Loss: Gluten Free Recipes for Celiac Disease, Gluten Sensitivities & Paleo Free Diets

Almond Flour Recipes for Optimal Health & Quick Weight Loss: Gluten Free Recipes for Celiac Disease, Gluten Sensitivities & Paleo Free Diets

Wheat Free Diet for Beginners: Lose Weight Quickly, Achieve Optimal Health & Feel Energized with Gluten Free Recipes for Celiac Disease, Gluten Sensitivities & Paleo Free Diets

Detox Diet Guide: Lose Weight Quickly, Achieve Optimal Health & Feel Energized Through the 10 Day Detox

Sugar Detox Guide for Beginners: Lose Weight Quickly, Achieve Optimal Health, Feel Energized & Eliminate Sugar Cravings Naturally

Ketogenic Diet Guide for Beginners: How to Achieve Rapid Weight Loss, Optimal Health & Unstoppable Energy with Ketogenic Diet Recipes

Anti Inflammatory Diet for Beginners: Lose Weight Fast, Optimize Health, Slow Aging, Fight Inflammation, Conquer Pain & Increase Energy with the Anti Inflammation Diet Recipes

One Last Thing...

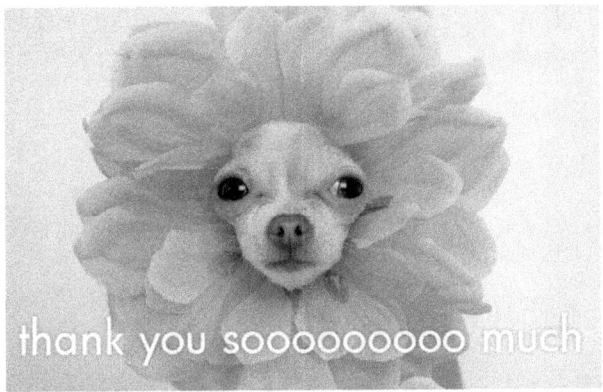

If you believe that this book is worth sharing, would you please take the time to let others know how it affected your life? If it turns out to make a difference in the lives of others, they will be forever grateful to you, as will I.

www.ingramcontent.com/pod-product-compliance
Lightning Source LLC
Chambersburg PA
CBHW070614290526
45790CB00002B/918